Allie's Asthma Adventures

Little Med Minds Series

Written By: Josephine Yalovitser and Christopher Kruglik
Illustrations By: Josephine Yalovitser

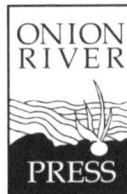

ONION
RIVER
PRESS

Burlington, Vermont

Onion River Press
89 Church Street
Burlington, VT 05401

info@onionriverpress.com
www.onionriverpress.com

ISBN: 978-1-966607-28-1
Library of Congress Control Number: 2025915940

We dedicate this book in memory of Dr. Laurence Coffin, a Vermont heart surgeon and painter whose creativity and accomplishments continue to inspire projects like this one. His legacy lives on through family and friends who carry on his mission to bridge arts and medicine, improving patient education and outcomes through creative and compassionate innovation.

With heartfelt thanks to Dr. Thomas Lahiri, whose wise guidance and kind support helped bring this story to life.

Little Med Minds Series: Allie's Asthma Adventures

Come join us as we explore the world of Allie's Asthma Adventures—a special edition from the *Little Med Minds* series! Follow Allie as she explores symptoms and triggers related to her asthma, what happens when she goes to her doctor's office to talk about difficulty breathing, and how her doctors help her feel better with an inhaler.

Little Med Minds is here to:

- Teach kids about their bodies and health in fun and easy ways
- Give kids superpowers like bravery and curiosity, so they can take an active role in their own care
- Answer questions that kids might have about hospitals, check-ups, and more
- Help turn scary moments, like doctor visits or procedures, into exciting learning adventures
- Build trust between children and their doctors
- Spark a love for medicine and science through memorable stories

In this adventure led by Allie, kids will:

- Learn how their lungs power playtime—and how asthma is just a "bump" in the road
- Discover how medications such as inhalers can help make their breathing easy
- See how doctors and families team up to tackle asthma together

For Parents & Caregivers:

This book is a tool to start conversations, ease worries, and empower your child. While Allie's journey teaches kids important lessons about their health, always consult your healthcare provider for medical advice.

Do you love learning with Allie?

Explore more *Little Med Minds* stories to grow your child's curiosity and confidence! Available where all books are sold.

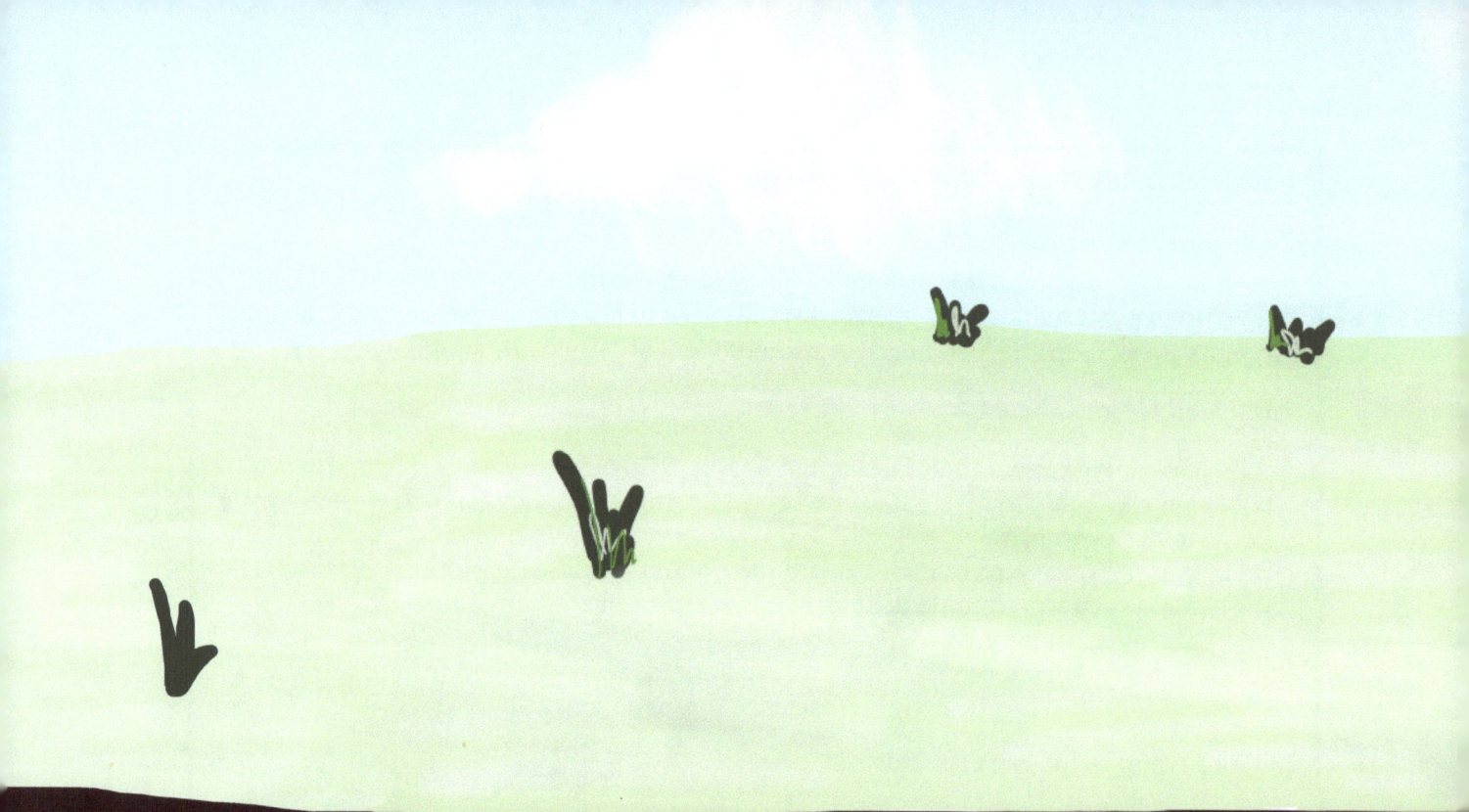

There once was a girl from a faraway town,

she had lots of animals and farmland around.

Her name was Allie and she was oh so cheery!

But when spring came around, things began to get dreary.

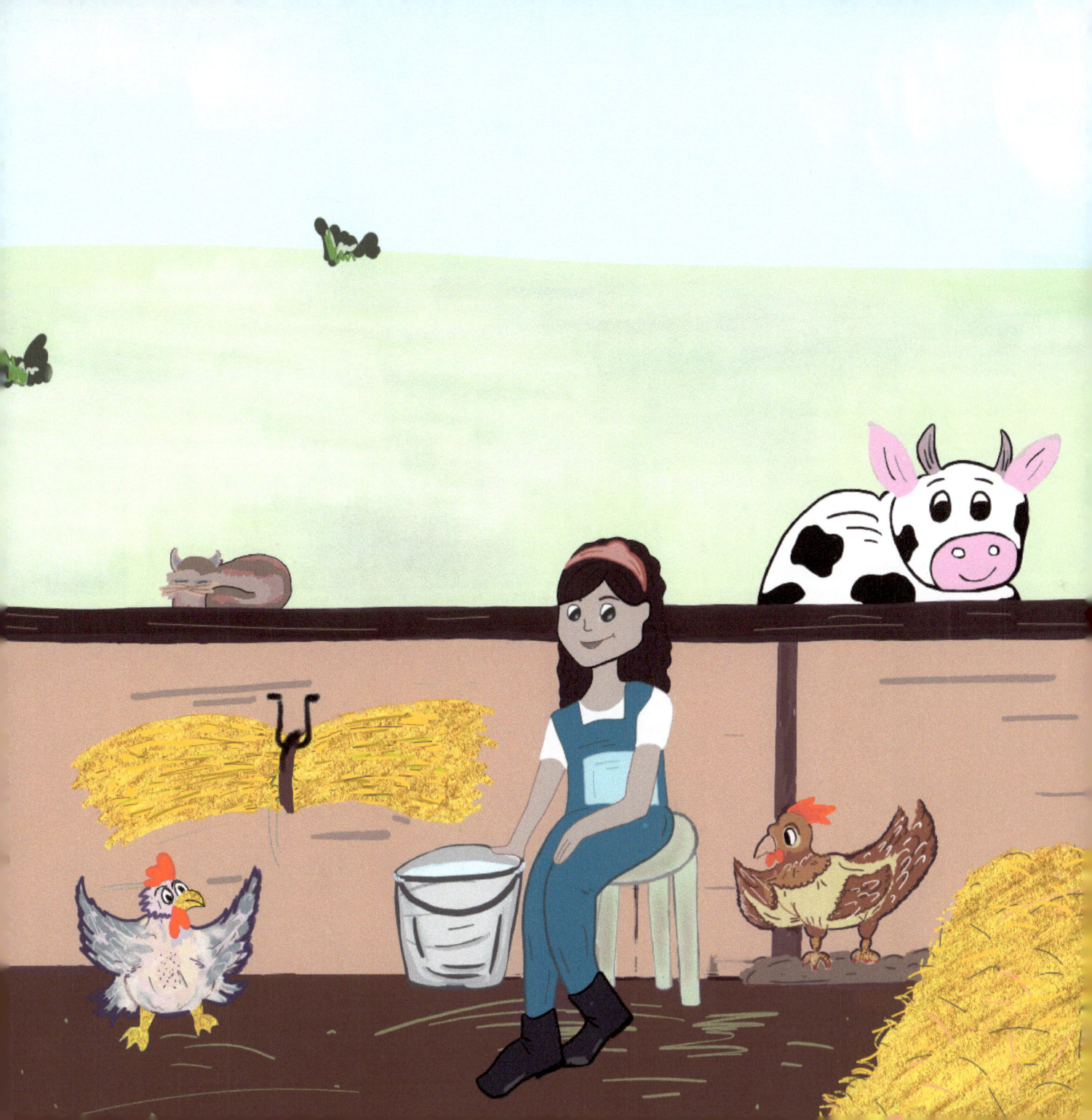

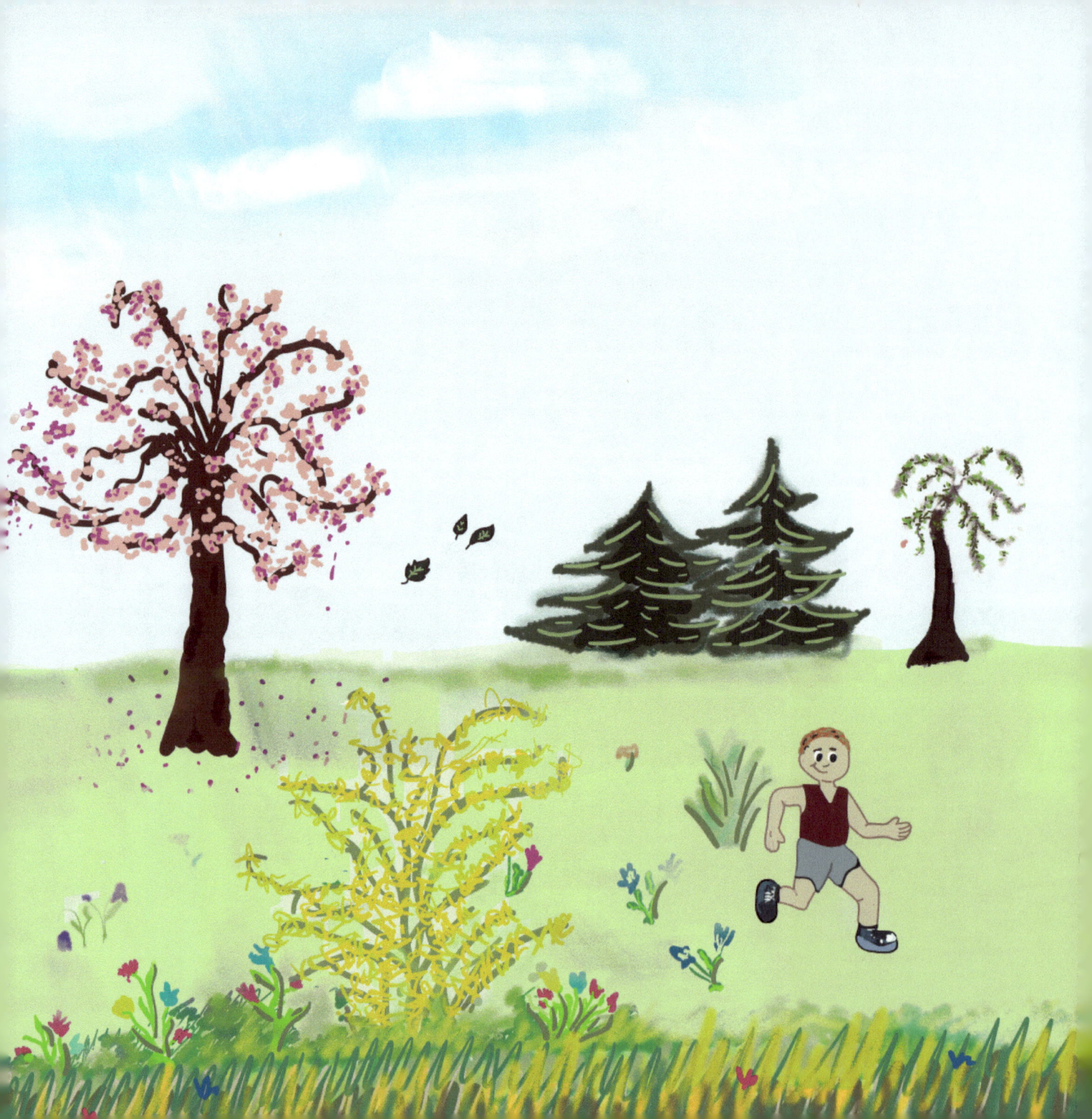

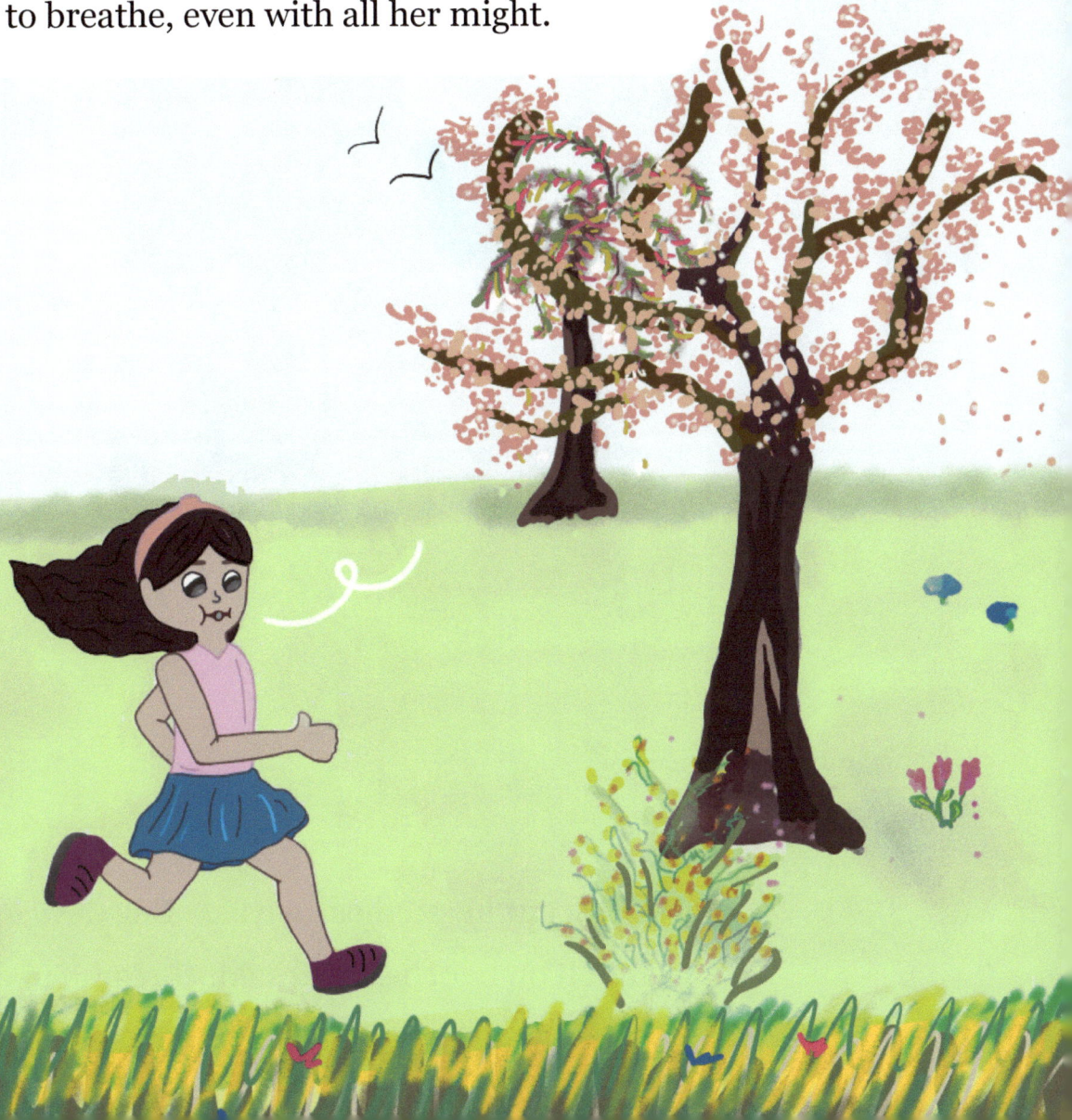

A few times at recess, she played "Duck, Duck, Goose!"

She ran super-fast, with her hair flying loose.

But all of a sudden her chest got real tight,

it was harder to breathe, even with all her might.

Allie went to the doctor she saw in her town,
and climbed onto the table with a slight frown.
The doc took a look, and gave a soft sigh,
"I'm sorry you've felt off, let's figure out why."

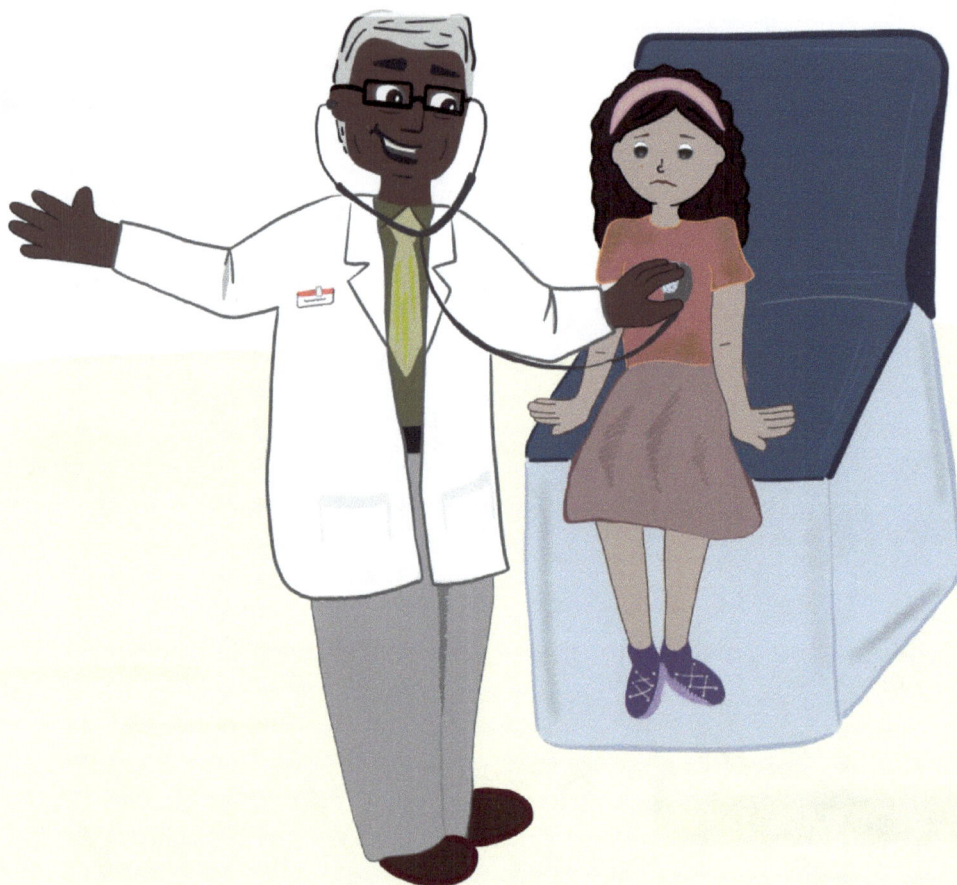

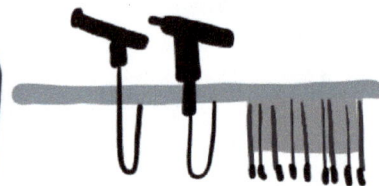

He took out his stethoscope listening device,
placed it on her chest and said, "Breathe in deeply twice."

"I hear lots of wheezing, high-pitched whistling sounds from deep in your chest where your two lungs are found.

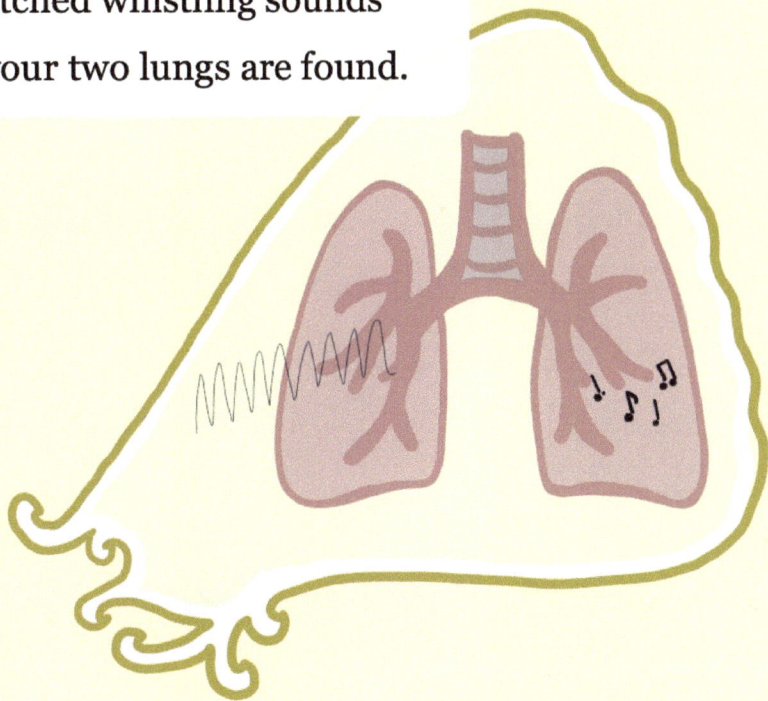

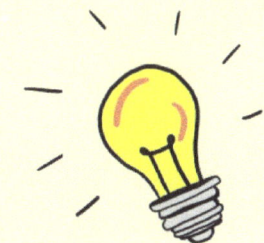

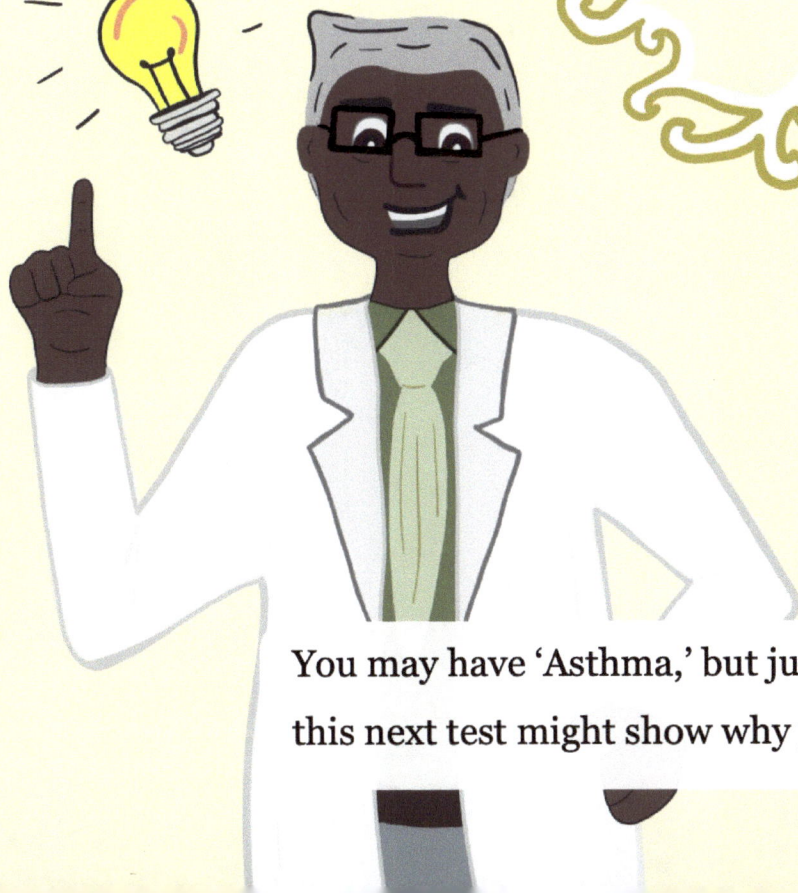

You may have 'Asthma,' but just to be certain, this next test might show why your chest has been hurtin'.

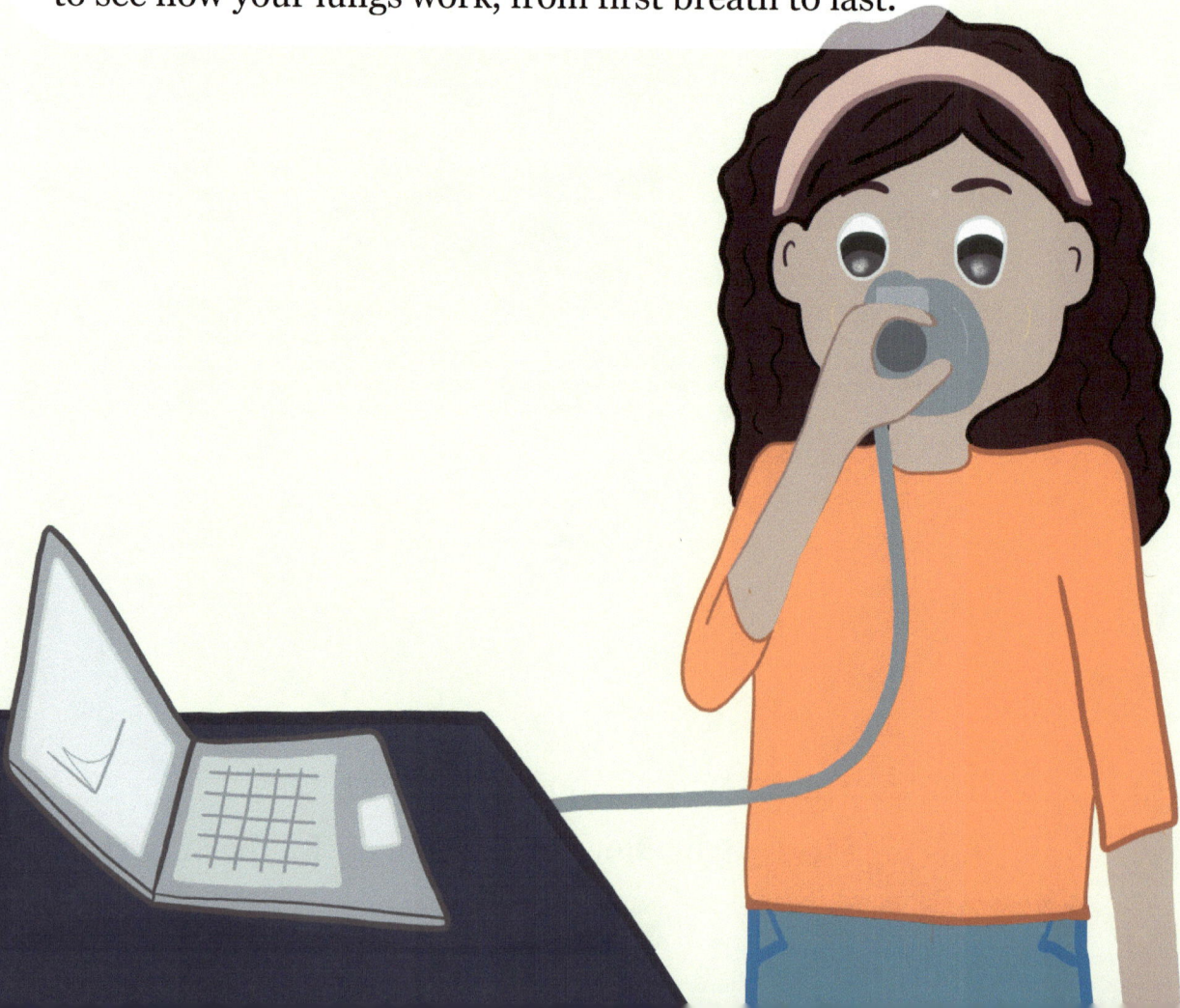

A "spirometer" gives us your breathing report,

In case that your lungs might need some support.

Breathe in real deep, fill up your airbag,

then blow it all out – go ahead, don't lag!

We measure the air that you push out real fast,

to see how your lungs work, from first breath to last.

Asthma has triggers both hidden and seen,
like cigarette smoke that makes air not so clean.
Viruses, exercise, even cold air,
can irritate airways and make asthma flare!

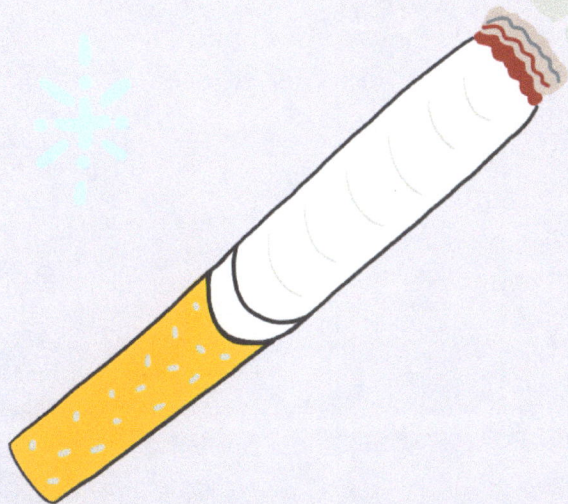
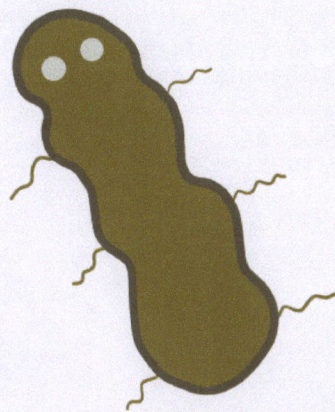
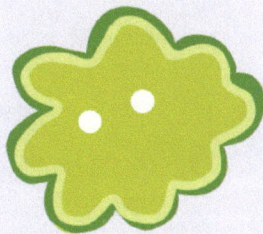
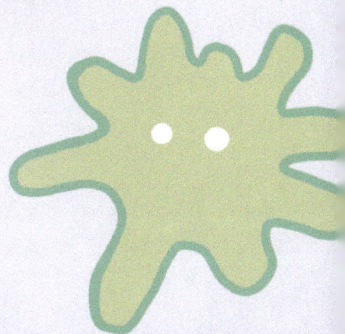

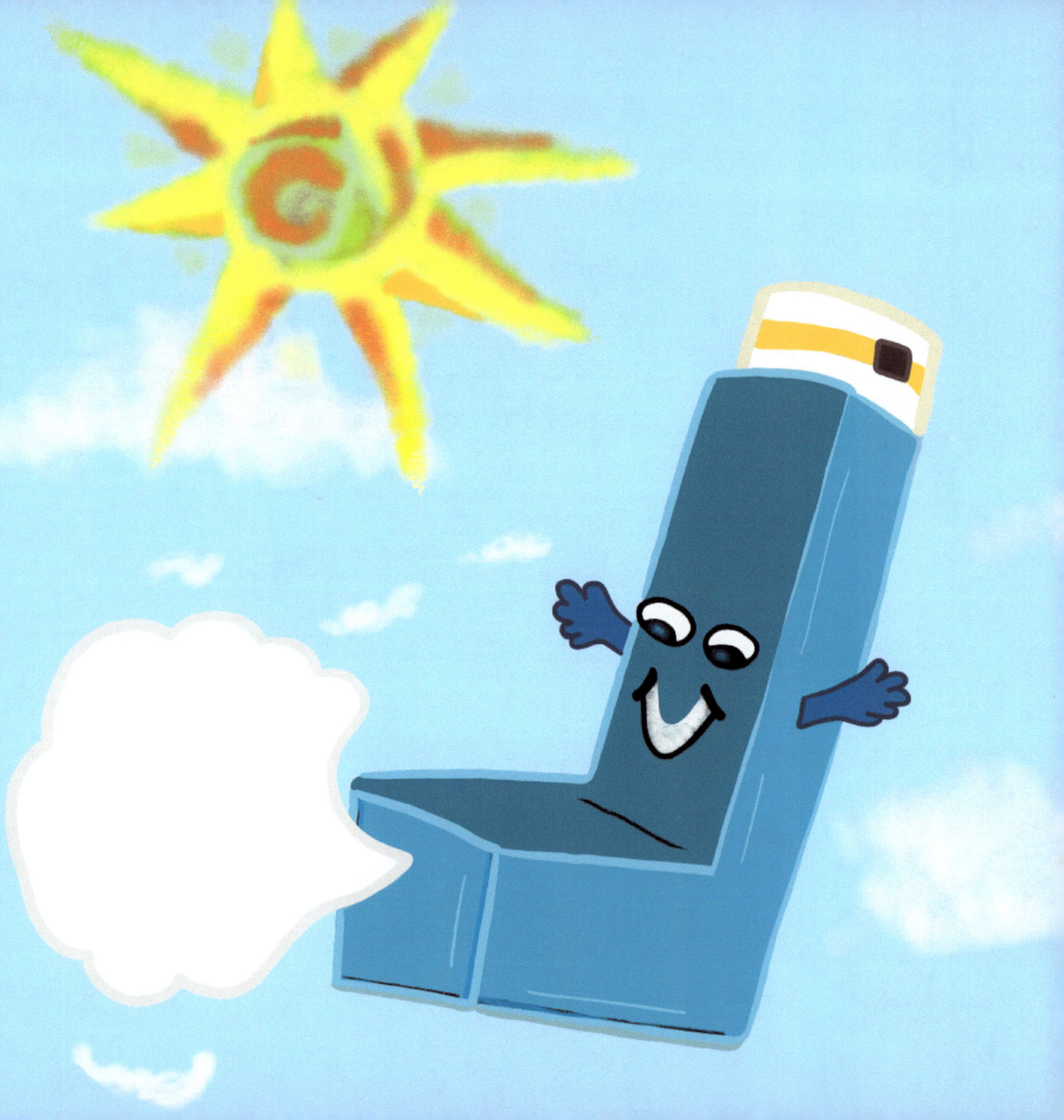

So here's an inhaler, a pretty neat tool,

to use when you're running or jumping at school.

Next time when you notice an 'asthma attack'

use the inhaler and stop it right in its tracks.

First, you breathe out as much as you can

while giving the canister a shake with your hand.

Then put the inhaler and spacer together—

with this handy tool you'll be feeling much better.

Place the mouthpiece gently right by your lips,

Press down on the button, and take in a deep sip.

The magic inside is called 'albuterol'
it relaxes lung muscles, both big and small!
It reduces swelling and clears out the goo,
so that you can breathe and no longer feel blue."

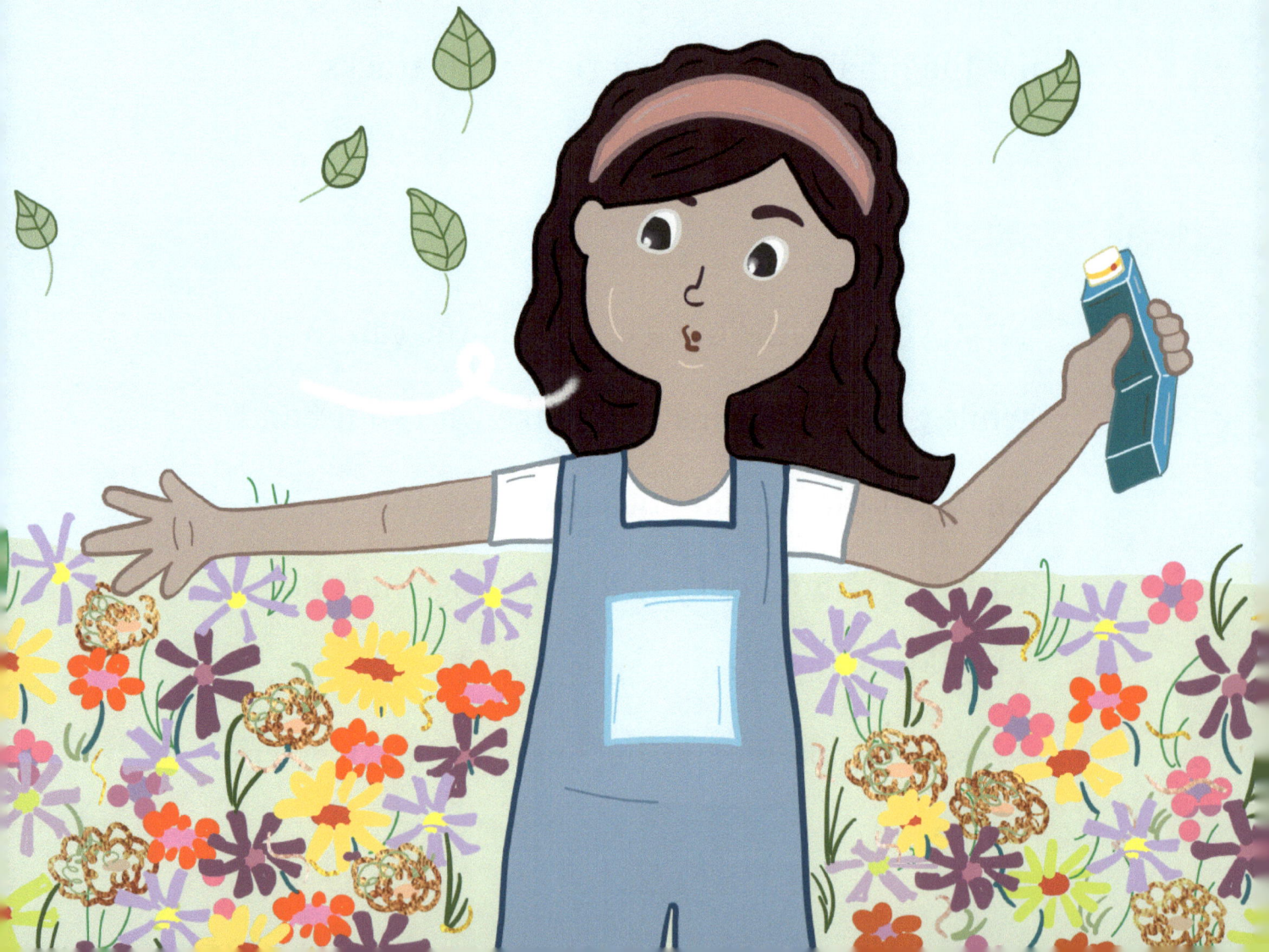

Even though Allie was using it right,

she still woke up coughing once a week in the night.

After a whole month, she started to fret,

so the doc said, "It looks like you need the next step."

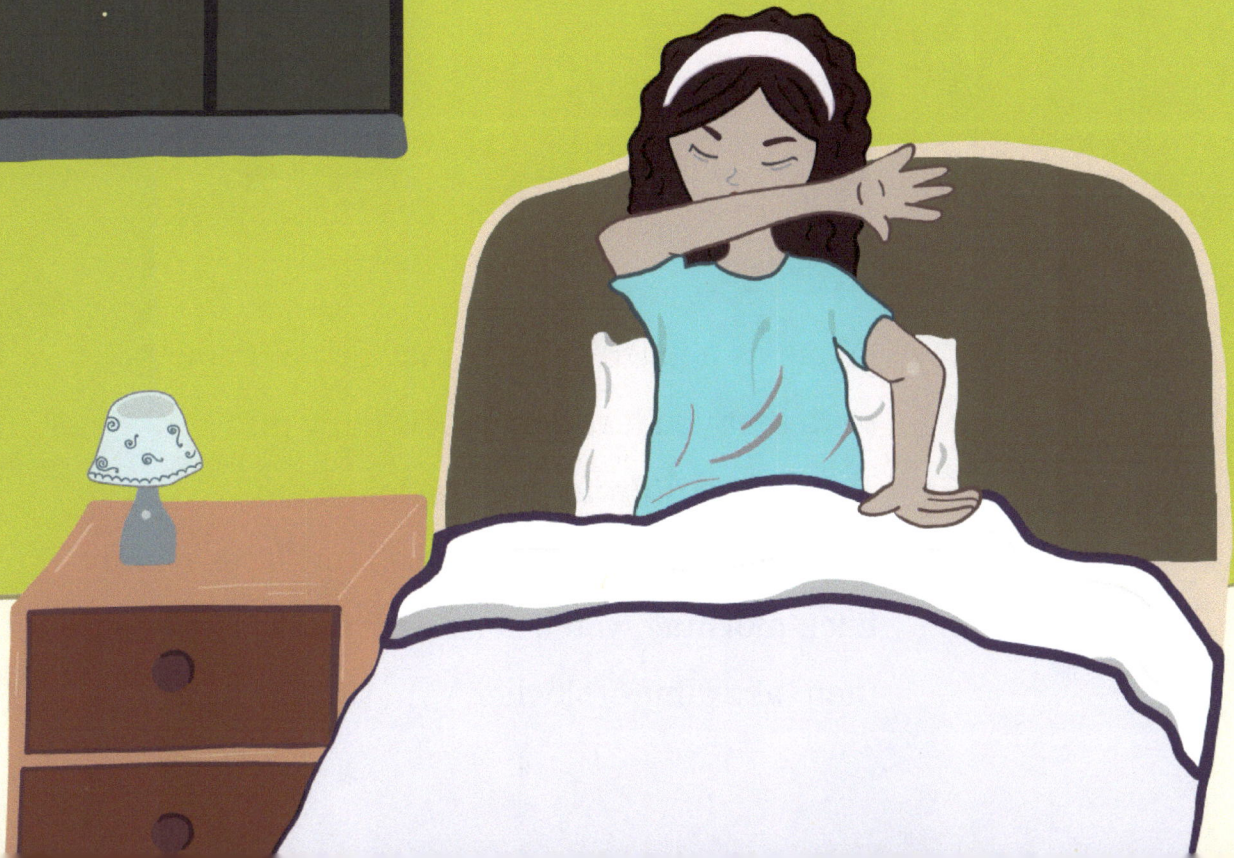

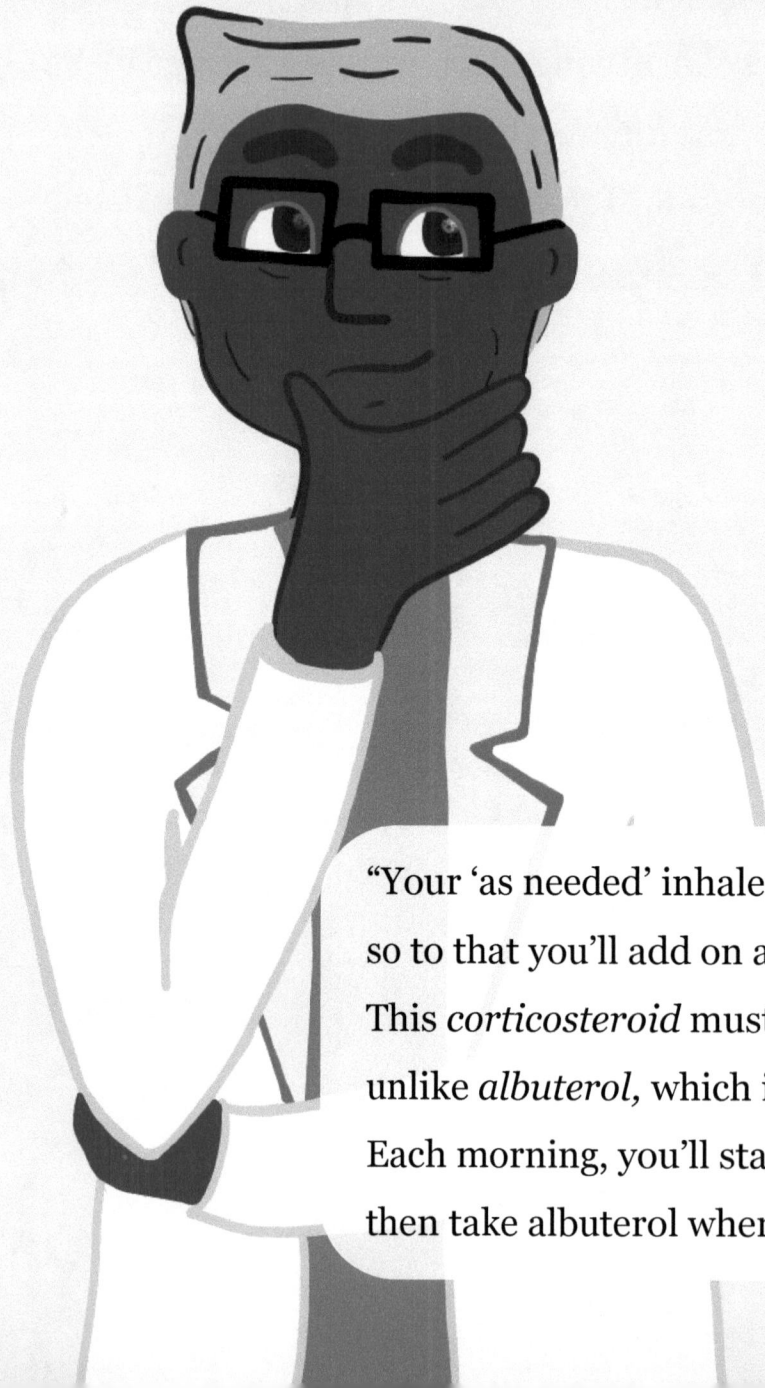

"Your 'as needed' inhaler may not be enough,
so to that you'll add on a new daily puff.
This *corticosteroid* must be taken daily,
unlike *albuterol,* which is used for flares mainly.
Each morning, you'll start with this special new med,
then take albuterol when gym time's ahead.

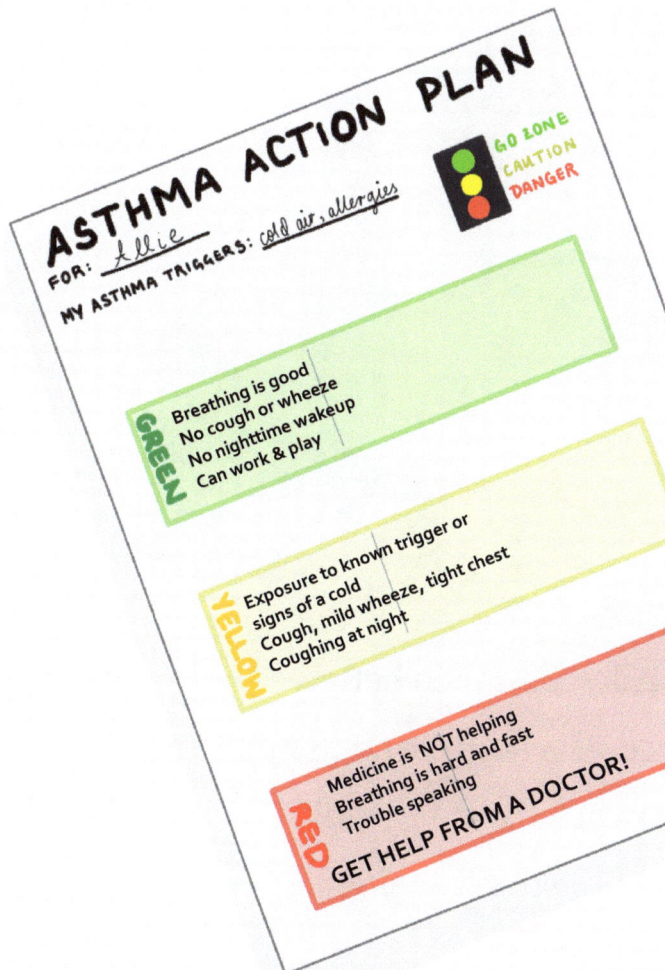

ASTHMA ACTION PLAN

FOR: _Allie_

MY ASTHMA TRIGGERS: _cold air, allergies_

GO ZONE
CAUTION
DANGER

GREEN
Breathing is good
No cough or wheeze
No nighttime wakeup
Can work & play

YELLOW
Exposure to known trigger or signs of a cold
Cough, mild wheeze, tight chest
Coughing at night

RED
Medicine is NOT helping
Breathing is hard and fast
Trouble speaking
GET HELP FROM A DOCTOR!

Green Zone means 'Go'

keep up your routine!

The daily meds help your lungs feel super clean.

Yellow Zone means 'Caution' when triggers appear,

use albuterol if wheezing feels ever so near.

Red Zone means 'Danger' don't wait or ignore

if your meds aren't helping and breathing's a chore.

With red you'll act fast—find adults right away

to get your lungs on track and make sure you're okay!

With this plan in hand, you're ready and aware

to manage your asthma with confidence and care!"

Show & Tell

MULTIPLICATION

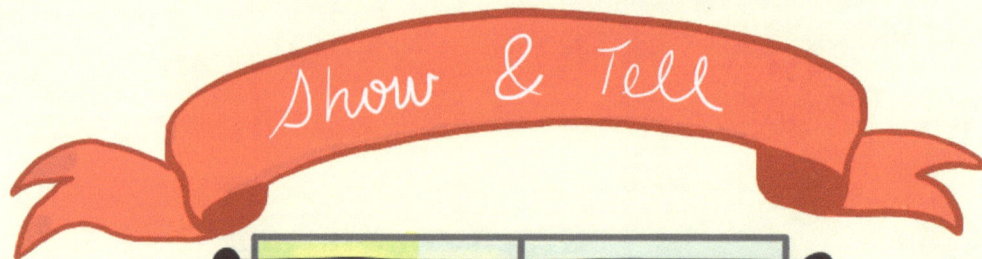

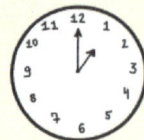

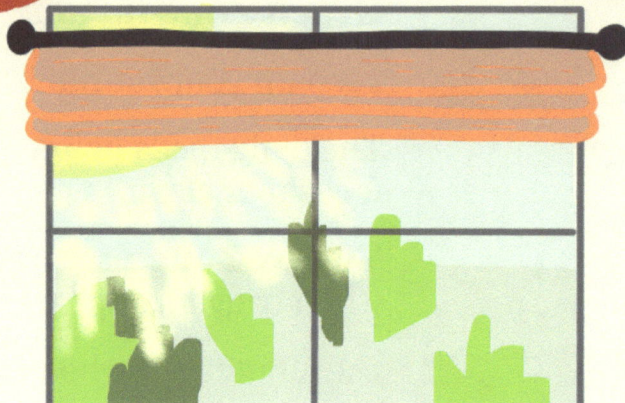

	1	2	3	4	5
1	1	2	3	4	5
2	2	4	6	8	10
3	3	6	9	12	15
4	4	8	12	16	20
5	5	10	15	20	25
6	6	12	18	24	30

The next year went by, and Allie felt much better.
She ran, jumped, and climbed—no matter the weather!
With her trusty inhaler, she won "Show and Tell"
and taught all her friends about asthma spells.

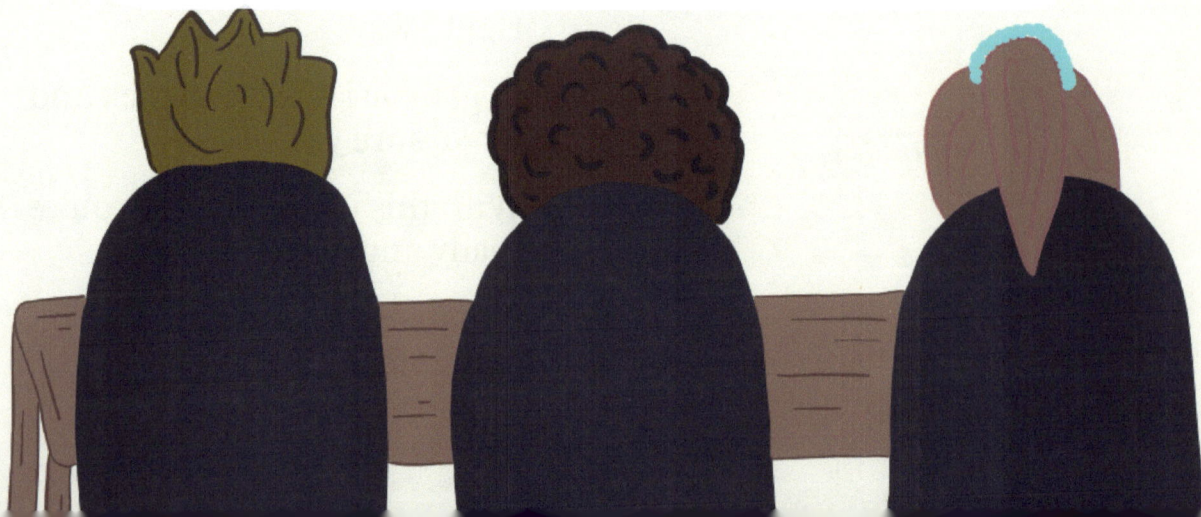

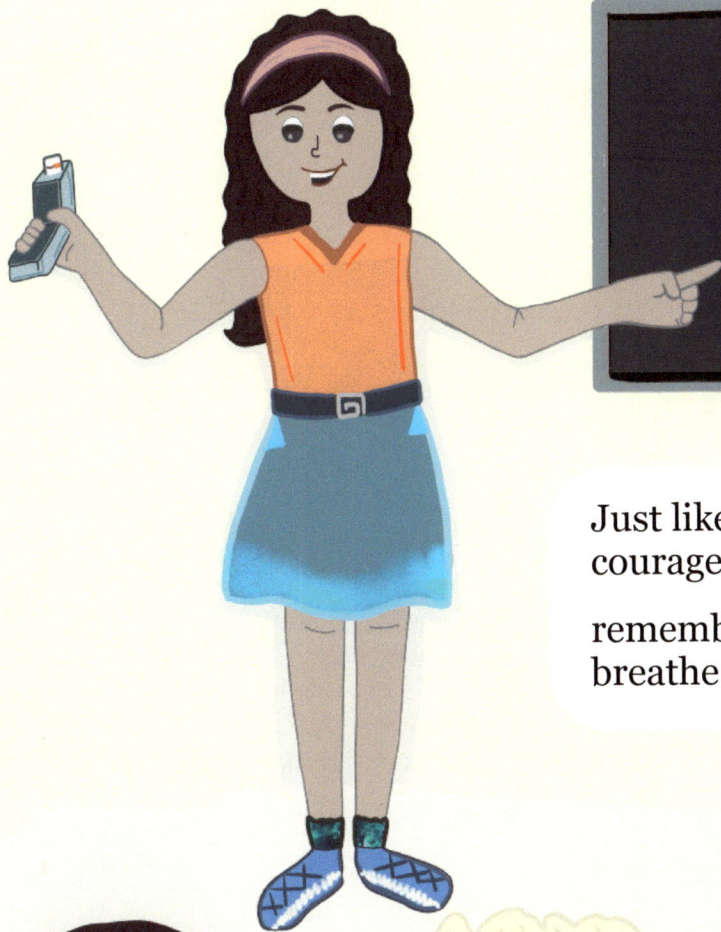

ASTHMA!

Just like Allie, who faced this with courage so true,

remember you've got the power to breathe easy, too!

ALLIE'S ASTHMA ADVENTURES MINI-QUIZ

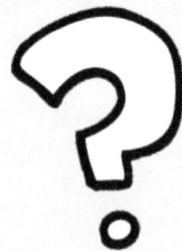

1. **What did Allie use to help her breathe before gym time?**
   a. A magic spell
   b. An albuterol inhaler
   c. A teddy bear

2. **What did the doctor use to listen to Allie's chest?**
   a. A listening device called a 'stethoscope'
   b. A magnifying glass
   c. A feather

3. **Which medication does Allie use as her "daily" inhaler?**
   a. Albuterol
   b. Corticosteroid
   c. Eat some ice cream

4. **What does the color "yellow" mean on Allie's Asthma Action Plan?**
   a. Caution! Use albuterol if symptoms or triggers appear
   b. Danger! Find a parent or doctor
   c. Sunshine! Go outside and play

5. **What did Allie teach her friends during "Show and Tell" at school?**
   a. How to ride a bike
   b. How to make a paper airplane
   c. About asthma and how to use an inhaler

Answers: B, A, B, A, C

Meet the Authors

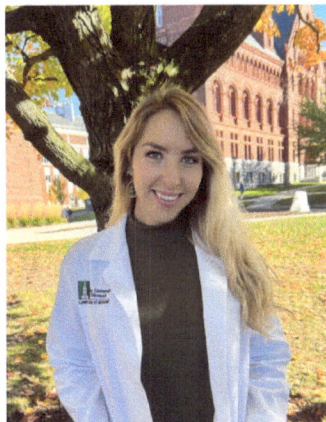

Josephine Yalovitser grew up in Westchester, New York, immersed in Russian culture as the child of immigrants. She discovered her love of the arts early on, with piano and singing at age four. Her work and original compositions have earned national and international recognition, with performances at prestigious venues including Carnegie Hall and Lincoln Center. She went on to study psychology and anthropology at Dartmouth College and will complete her medical degree from the University of Vermont College of Medicine in 2026. Passionate about the intersection of medicine and the arts, Josephine strives to bring creativity, empathy, and a holistic perspective to patient care. Whether through music, medicine, or storytelling, she is committed to healing that honors the full human experience.

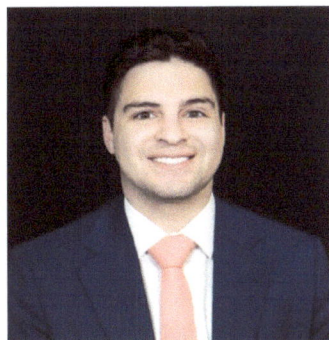

Born in New Haven, Connecticut, in 1997, Christopher Kruglik grew up in the small town of Northford, Connecticut, with his mother and father, two sisters, and two brothers. He went on to receive his Bachelor of Science degree in Biochemistry at the University of Vermont, as well as his Master of Medical Sciences and Master of Public Health. As of 2025, Christopher is currently enrolled in his last year of medical school at the Larner College of Medicine at the University of Vermont. Christopher's clinical interests lie within the sector of the public health realm, pediatrics, and surgery. He is excited to be able to share the *Little Med Minds* book series with his co-author and illustrator to help make children more comfortable and prepared when seeing their physician or getting ready for a surgical procedure.

www.ingramcontent.com/pod-product-compliance
Lightning Source LLC
Chambersburg PA
CBHW061147030426

42335CB00002B/142